My Pegan Breakfast Diet Cookbook

Easy and Tasty Recipes for your Paleo and Vegan Breakfast

Kimberly Solis

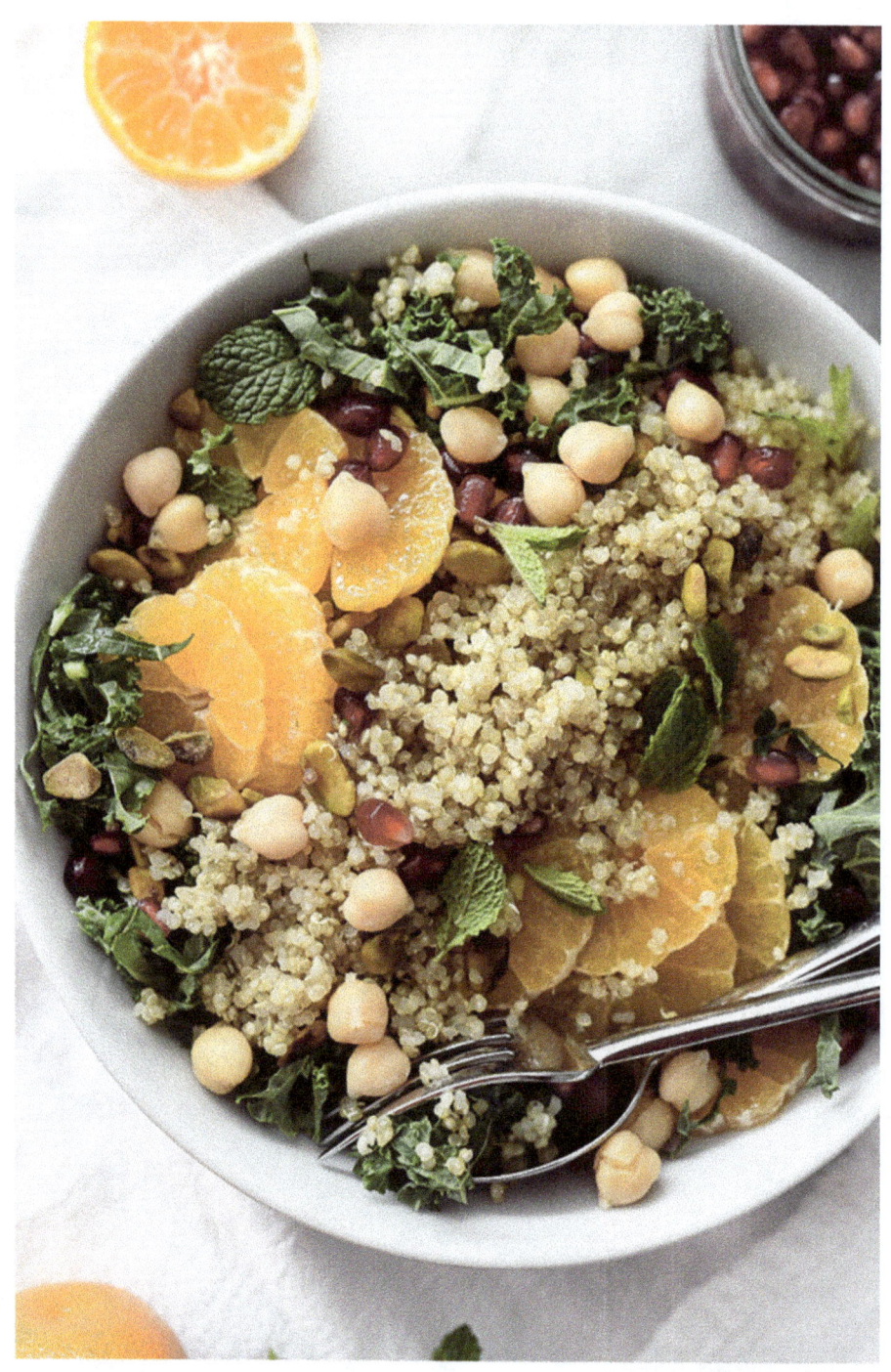

© **copyright 2021 – all rights reserved.**

the content contained within this book may not be reproduced, duplicated or transmitted without direct written permission from the author or the publisher.

under no circumstances will any blame or legal responsibility be held against the publisher, or author, for any damages, reparation, or monetary loss due to the information contained within this book. either directly or indirectly.

legal notice:

this book is copyright protected. this book is only for personal use. you cannot amend, distribute, sell, use, quote or paraphrase any part, or the content within this book, without the consent of the author or publisher.

disclaimer notice:

please note the information contained within this document is for educational and entertainment purposes only. all effort has been executed to present accurate, up to date, and reliable, complete information. no warranties of any kind are declared or implied. readers acknowledge that the author is not engaging in the rendering of legal, financial, medical or professional advice. the content within this book has been derived from various sources. please consult a licensed professional before attempting any techniques outlined in this book.

by reading this document, the reader agrees that under no circumstances is the author responsible for any losses, direct or indirect, which are incurred as a result of the use of information contained within this document, including, but not limited to, — errors, omissions, or inaccuracies.

Table of Contents

GREEN BREAKFAST SMOOTHIE 6
WARM MAPLE AND CINNAMON QUINOA 8
BLUEBERRY AND CHIA SMOOTHIE 10
APPLE AND CINNAMON OATMEAL 12
SPICED ORANGE BREAKFAST COUSCOUS 14
BROILED GRAPEFRUIT WITH CINNAMON PITAS 16
BREAKFAST PARFAITS 18
ORANGE FRENCH TOAST 20
PUMPKIN PANCAKES 22
SWEET POTATO AND KALE HASH 24
SAVORY OATMEAL PORRIDGE 26
PUMPKIN STEEL-CUT OATS 28
CINNAMON AND SPICE OVERNIGHT OATS 30
BARLEY BREAKFAST BOWL 32
SWEET POTATO AND BLACK BEAN HASH 34
SMOOTHIE BREAKFAST BOWL 36
TORTILLA BREAKFAST CASSEROLE 38
TOFU-SPINACH SCRAMBLE 40
SAVORY PANCAKES 42
QUINOA BREAKFAST PORRIDGE 44
GRAPES AND GREEN TEA SMOOTHIE 46
MANGO AND KALE SMOOTHIE 48
POMEGRANATE SMOOTHIE 50
COCONUT WATER SMOOTHIE 52
APPLE, BANANA, AND BERRY SMOOTHIE 53
BERRY GINGER ZING SMOOTHIE 55
DRAGON FRUIT SMOOTHIE BOWL 57
CHOCOLATE SMOOTHIE BOWL 59
ZUCCHINI AND BLUEBERRY SMOOTHIE 61

- Hot Pink Beet Smoothie 63
- Chickpea Flour Frittata 65
- Potato Pancakes 68
- Chocolate Chip Pancakes 70
- Turmeric Steel-Cut Oats 72
- Vegetable Pancakes 75
- Banana and Chia Pudding 78
- Tofu Scramble 81
- Pumpkin Spice Oatmeal 84
- Peanut Butter Bites 86
- Maple and Cinnamon Overnight Oats 88
- Breakfast Tomato and Eggs 90
- Breakfast Paleo Muffins 92
- Paleo Banana Pancakes 94
- Breakfast Eggs 96
- Plantain Pancakes 98
- Sweet Potato Waffles 100
- Eggplant French Toast 102
- Orange and Dates Granola 104

Green Breakfast Smoothie

Preparation Time: 10 minutes

Cooking time: 0 minutes

Servings: 2

Ingredients:
- 1/2 Banana, sliced
- 2 cups spinach
- 1 cup sliced berries of your choosing, fresh or frozen
- 1 orange, peeled and cut into segments
- 1 cup unsweetened nondairy milk
- 1 cup ice

Directions:
1. In a blender, combine all the ingredients.
2. Starting with the blender on low speed, begin blending the smoothie, gradually increasing blender speed until smooth. Serve immediately.

Nutrition:

Calories: 208;

Fat: 8g;

Protein: 14g;

Carbohydrates: 22g;

Fiber: 7g;

Sugar: 1g;

Sodium: 596mg

Warm Maple and Cinnamon Quinoa

Preparation Time: 5 minutes

Cooking time: 15 minutes

Servings: 4

Ingredients:
- 1 cup unsweetened nondairy milk
- 1 cup water
- 1 cup quinoa, rinsed
- 1 teaspoon cinnamon
- 1/4 cup chopped pecans
- 2 tablespoons pure maple syrup or agave
-

Directions:
1. Bring the almond milk, water, and quinoa to a boil. Lower the heat to medium-low and cover. Cook gently until the quinoa softens, about 15 minutes.
2. Turn off the heat and allow sitting, covered, for 5 minutes. Stir in the cinnamon, pecans, and syrup. Serve hot.

Nutrition:

Calories: 110;

Fat: 9g;

Protein: 15g;

Carbohydrates: 25g;

Fiber: 7g;

Sugar: 4g;

Sodium: 210mg

Blueberry and Chia Smoothie

Preparation Time: 10 minutes
Cooking time: 0 minutes
Servings: 2

Ingredients:
- 2 tablespoons chia seeds
- 2 cups unsweetened nondairy milk
- 2 cups blueberries, fresh or frozen
- 2 tablespoons pure maple syrup or agave
- 2 tablespoons cocoa powder

Directions:
1. Blend together the soaked chia seeds, almond milk, blueberries, maple syrup, and cocoa powder and blend until smooth. Serve immediately

Nutrition:
Calories: 100;
Fat: 18g;
Protein: 19g;
Carbohydrates: 20g;
Fiber: 9g;
Sugar: 4g;

Sodium: 500mg

Apple and Cinnamon Oatmeal

Preparation Time: 5 minutes

Cooking time: 15 minutes

Servings: 4

Ingredients:
- 1/4 cups apple cider
- 1 apple, peeled, cored, and chopped
- 2/3 cup rolled oats
- 1 teaspoon ground cinnamon
- 1 tablespoon pure maple syrup

Directions:
1. Take the apple cider to a boil over medium-high heat. Stir in the apple, oats, and cinnamon.
2. Bring the cereal to a boil and turn down heat to low. Simmer until the oatmeal thickens, 3 to 4 minutes. Spoon into two bowls and sweeten with maple syrup, if using. Serve hot.

Nutrition:

Calories: 110;

Fat: 9g;

Protein: 15g;

Carbohydrates: 25g;

Fiber: 7g;

Sugar: 4g;

Sodium: 210mg

Spiced Orange Breakfast Couscous

Preparation Time: 5 minutes
Cooking time: 15 minutes
Servings: 4

Ingredients:
- 3 cups orange juice
- 1.1/2 cups couscous
- 1 teaspoon ground cinnamon
- 1/4 teaspoon ground cloves
- 1/2 cup dried fruit
- 1/2 cup chopped almonds

Directions:
1. Take the orange juice to a boil. Add the couscous, cinnamon, and cloves and remove from heat. Shield the pan and allow sitting until the -couscous softens.
2. Fluff the couscous and stir in the dried fruit and nuts. Serve -immediately. Pecans and syrup. Serve hot.

Nutrition:

Calories: 110;

Fat: 9g;

Protein: 15g;

Carbohydrates: 25g;

Fiber: 7g;

Sugar: 4g;

Sodium: 210mg

Broiled Grapefruit with Cinnamon Pitas

Preparation Time: 5 minutes

Cooking time: 15 minutes

Servings: 4

Ingredients:
- 2 whole-wheat pitas cut into wedges
- 2 tablespoons coconut oil, melted
- 1 tablespoon ground cinnamon
- 2 tablespoons brown sugar
- 1 grapefruit, halved
- 2 tablespoons pure maple syrup or agave

Directions:
1. Preheat the oven to 375°F. Line a baking sheet with parchment paper.
2. Spread pita wedges in a single layer on a baking sheet and brush with melted coconut oil.
3. In a small bowl, combine the cinnamon and brown sugar and sprinkle over the pita wedges.

4. Bake in preheated oven until the wedges are crisp, about 8 minutes. Transfer the pita wedges to a plate and set aside.
5. Turn the oven to broil. Drip the maple syrup over the top of the grapefruit, if using. Broil until the syrup bubbles and begins to crystallize, 3 to 5 minutes. Serve immediately.

Nutrition:

Calories: 115;

Fat: 19g;

Protein: 25g;

Carbohydrates: 35g;

Fiber: 17g;

Sugar: 14g;

Sodium: 210mg

Breakfast Parfaits

Preparation Time: 5 minutes
Cooking time: 15 minutes
Servings: 4

Ingredients:
- One 14-ounce cans coconut milk, refrigerated overnight
- 1 cup granola
- 1/2 cup walnuts
- 1 cup sliced strawberries or other seasonal berries

Directions:
1. Pour off the canned coconut-milk liquid and retain the solids.
2. In two parfait glasses, layer the coconut-milk solids, granola, walnuts, and -strawberries. Serve immediately.

Nutrition:
Calories: 125;
Fat: 9g;
Protein: 15g;
Carbohydrates: 35g;

Fiber: 17g;

Sugar: 18g;

Sodium: 310mg

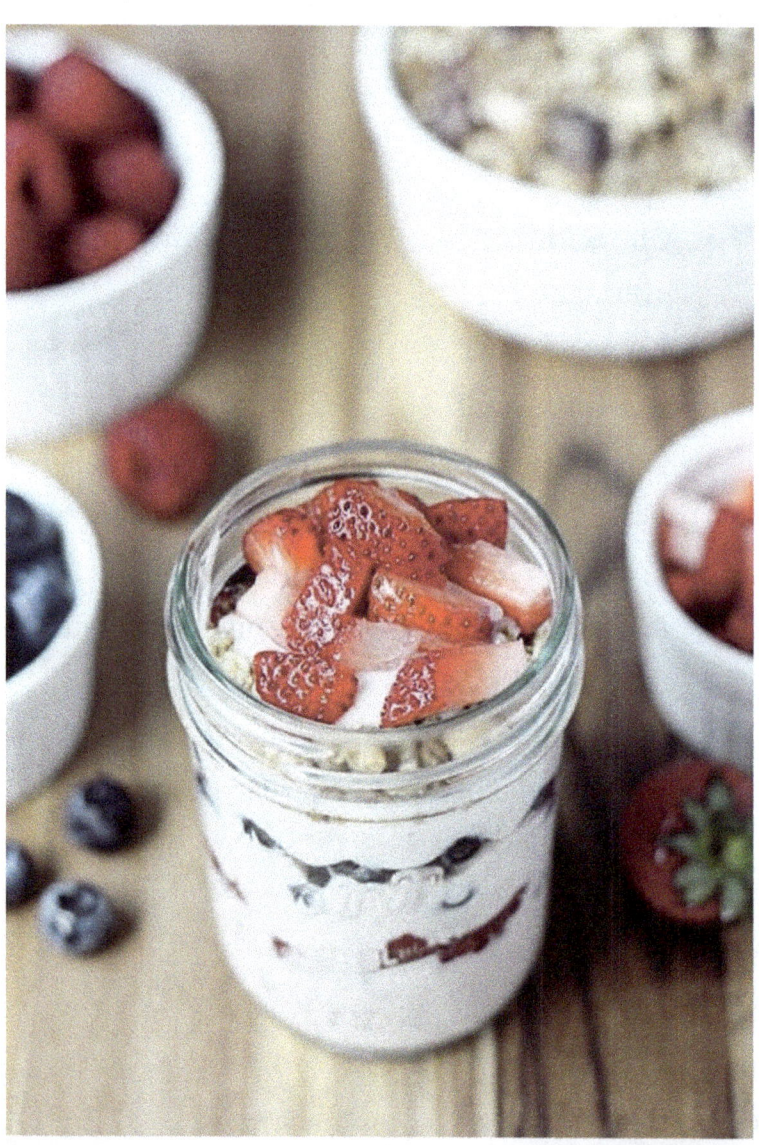

Orange French toast

Preparation Time: 5 minutes
Cooking time: 15 minutes
Servings: 4

Ingredients:
- 3 very ripe bananas
- 1 cup unsweetened nondairy milk
- Zest and juice of 1 orange
- 1 teaspoon ground cinnamon
- 1/4 teaspoon grated nutmeg
- 4 slices French bread
- 1 tablespoon coconut oil

Directions:
1. Blend the bananas, almond milk, orange juice and zest, cinnamon, and nutmeg and blend until smooth. Dip the bread in the mixture for 5 minutes on each side.
2. While the bread soaks, heat a griddle or sauté pan over medium-high heat. Melt the coconut oil in the pan and swirl to coat. Cook the bread slices until golden brown on both sides, about 5 minutes each. Serve immediately.

Nutrition:

Calories: 113;

Fat: 19g;

Protein: 25g;

Carbohydrates: 85g;

Fiber: 19g;

Sugar: 18g;

Sodium: 320mg

Pumpkin Pancakes

Preparation Time: 5 minutes

Cooking time: 15 minutes

Servings: 4

Ingredients:
- 2 cups unsweetened almond milk
- 1 teaspoon apple cider vinegar
- 2.1/2 cups whole-wheat flour
- 2 tablespoons baking powder
- 1/2 teaspoon baking soda
- 1 teaspoon sea salt
- 1 teaspoon pumpkin pie
- 1/2 cup canned pumpkin purée
- 1 cup water
- 1 tablespoon coconut oil

Directions:
1. Dip together the flour, baking powder, baking soda, salt and pumpkin pie spice.
2. In another large bowl, combine the almond milk mixture, pumpkin purée, and water, whisking to mix well.

3. Add the wet ingredients to the dry ingredients and fold together until the dry -ingredients are just moistened. You will still have a few streaks of flour in the bowl.
4. In a nonstick pan or griddle over medium-high heat, melt the coconut oil and swirl to coat. Pour the batter into the pan 1/4 cup at a time and cook until the pancakes are browned, about 5 minutes per side. Serve immediately.

Nutrition:

Calories: 113;

Fat: 19g;

Protein: 25g;

Carbohydrates: 85g;

Fiber: 19g;

Sugar: 18g;

Sodium: 320mg

Sweet Potato and Kale Hash

Preparation Time: 10 minutes
Cooking time: 15 minutes
Servings: 2

Ingredients:

- 1 sweet potato
- 2 tablespoons olive oil
- 1/2 onion, chopped
- 1 carrot, peeled and chopped
- 2 garlic cloves, minced
- 1/2 teaspoon dried thyme
- 1 cup chopped kale
- Sea salt
- Freshly ground black pepper

Directions:

1. Pierce the sweet potato and microwave on high until soft, about 5 minutes. Remove from the microwave and cut into 1/4-inch cubes.
2. In a large nonstick sauté pan, heat the olive oil over medium-high heat. Add the onion and carrot and cook until softened, about 5 minutes. Attach the

garlic and thyme until the garlic is fragrant, about 30 seconds.

3. Add the sweet potatoes and cook until the potatoes begin to brown, about 7 -minutes. Add the kale and cook just until it wilts, 1 to 2 minutes. Season with salt and pepper. Serve immediately.

Nutrition:

Calories: 125;

Fat: 9g;

Protein: 15g;

Carbohydrates: 35g;

Fiber: 17g;

Sugar: 18g;

Sodium: 310mg

Savory Oatmeal Porridge

Preparation Time: 5 minutes

Cooking time: 20 minutes

Servings: 4

Ingredients:

- 2 1/2 cups vegetable broth
- 2 1/2 cups milk
- 1/2 cup steel-cut oats
- 1 tablespoon faro
- 1/2 cup slivered almonds
- 1/4 cup nutritional yeast
- 2 cups old-fashioned rolled oats
- 1/2 teaspoon salt (optional)

Directions:

1. Take the broth and almond milk to a boil. Add the oats, faro, almond slivers, and nutritional yeast. Cook over medium-high heat for 20 minutes, stirring occasionally.
2. Add the rolled oats and cook for another 5 minutes, until creamy. Stir in the salt (if using).
3. Divide into 4 single-serving containers. Let cool before sealing the lids.

Nutrition:

Calories: 152;

Fat: 16g;

Protein: 35g;

Carbohydrates: 55g;

Fiber: 25g;

Sugar: 18g;

Sodium: 245mg

Pumpkin Steel-Cut Oats

Preparation Time: 15 minutes

Cooking time: 25 minutes

Servings: 4

Ingredients:
- 3 cups water
- 1 cup steel-cut oats
- 1/2 cup canned pumpkin purée
- 1/4 cup pumpkin seeds (pipits)
- 2 tablespoons maple syrup
- Pinch salt

Directions:
1. Whip and reduce the heat to low. Simmer until the oats are soft, 20 to 30 minutes, continuing to stir occasionally.
2. Stir in the pumpkin purée and continue cooking on low for 3 to 5 minutes longer. Stir in the pumpkin seeds and maple syrup, and season with the salt.
3. Divide the oatmeal into 4 single-serving containers. Let cool before sealing the lids.

Nutrition:

Calories: 132;

Fat: 19;

Protein: 4535g;

Carbohydrates: 75g;

Fiber: 73; g

Sugar: 15; g

Sodium: 345mg

Cinnamon and Spice Overnight Oats

Preparation Time: 15 minutes

Cooking time: 20 minutes

Servings: 3

Ingredients:
- 2.1/2 cups old-fashioned rolled oats
- 5 tablespoons pumpkin seeds (pipits)
- 5 tablespoons chopped pecans
- 5 cups unsweetened plant-based milk
- 21/2 teaspoons maple syrup or agave syrup
- 1/2 to 1 teaspoon salt
- 1/2 to 1 teaspoon ground cinnamon
- 1/2 to 1 teaspoon ground ginger

Directions:
1. Line up 5 wide-mouth pint jars. In each jar, combine 1/2 cup of oats, 1 tablespoon of pumpkin seeds, 1 tablespoon of pecans, 1 cup of plant-based milk, 1/2 teaspoon of maple syrup, 1 pinch of salt, 1 pinch of cinnamon, and 1 pinch of ginger.

2. Stir the ingredients in each jar. Close the jars tightly with lids. To serve, top with fresh fruit (if using).

Nutrition:

Calories: 124;

Fat: 1927

Protein: 35g;

Carbohydrates: 80;

Fiber: 65 g

Sugar: 18 g

Sodium: 276

Barley Breakfast Bowl

Preparation Time: 5 minutes

Cooking time: 15minutes

Servings: 4

Ingredients:
- 1.1/2 cups pearl barley
- 3.3/4 cups water
- Large pinch salt
- 1.1/2 cups dried cranberries
- 3 cups sweetened vanilla plant-based milk
- 2 tablespoons slivered almonds (optional)

Directions:
1. Put the barley, water, and salt. Bring to a boil.
2. Divide the barley into 6 jars or single-serving storage containers. Attached the 1/4 cup of dried cranberries to each. Pour 1/2 cup of plant-based milk into each. Attached the 1 teaspoon of slivered almonds (if using) to each. Close the jars tightly with lids.

Nutrition:

Calories: 109;

Fat: 15g;

Protein: 24g;

Carbohydrates: 32g;

Fiber: 8g;

Sugar: 1g;

Sodium: 466mg

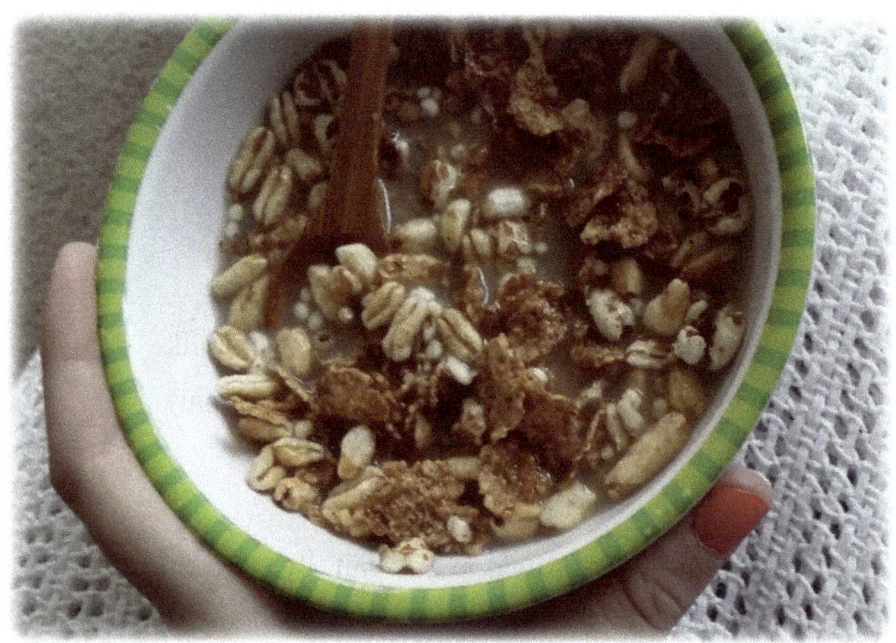

Sweet Potato and Black Bean Hash

Preparation Time: 10 minutes
Cooking time: 20minutes
Servings: 6

Ingredients:

- 1 teaspoon extra-virgin olive oil or 3 teaspoons vegetable broth
- 1 large sweet yellow onion, diced
- 2 teaspoons minced garlic (about 2 cloves)
- 1 large sweet potato, unpeeled, diced into ¾-inch pieces
- 2 teaspoons ground cumin
- 1 teaspoon dried oregano
- 1 (14.5-ounce) can black beans, rinsed and drained
- 1/4 teaspoon salt
- 1/4 teaspoon freshly ground black pepper

Directions:

1. In large skillet over medium-high heat, heat the olive oil. Attach the onion and garlic and cook for 5 minutes, stirring frequently.

2. Add the sweet potatoes, cumin, and oregano. Stir and cook for another 5 minutes. Cover the skillet, reduce the heat to low, and cook for 15 minutes.
3. After 15 minutes, increase the heat to medium-high and stir in the black beans, salt (if using), and pepper. Cook for another 5 minutes.
4. Divide evenly among 6 single-serving containers. Let cool before sealing the lids.

Nutrition:

Calories: 209;

Fat: 12g;

Protein: 34g;

Carbohydrates: 22g;

Fiber: 8g;

Sugar: 1g;

Sodium: 466mg

Smoothie Breakfast Bowl

Preparation Time: 10 minutes

Cooking time: 20minutes

Servings: 4

Ingredients:

- 4 bananas, peeled
- 1 cup dragon fruit or fruit of choice
- 1 cup Baked Granola
- 2 cups fresh berries
- 1/2 cup slivered almonds
- 4 cups plant-based milk

Directions:

1. Open 4 quart-size, freezer-safe bags, and layer in the following order: 1 banana (halved or sliced) and 1/4 cup dragon fruit.
2. Into 4 small jelly jars, layer in the following order: 1/4 cup granola, 1/2 cup berries, and 2 tablespoons slivered almonds.
3. To serve, take a frozen bag of bananas and dragon fruit and transfer to a blender. Add 1 cup of plant-based milk, and blend until smooth. Pour into a bowl. Add the contents of 1 jar of granola, berries, and

almonds over the top of the smoothie, and serve with a spoon.

Nutrition:

Calories: 109;

Fat: 12g;

Protein: 24g;

Carbohydrates: 24g;

Fiber: 8g;

Sugar: 5g;

Sodium: 366mg

Tortilla Breakfast Casserole

Preparation Time: 20 minutes

Cooking time: 20minutes

Servings: 4

Ingredients:
- 1 recipe Tofu-Spinach Scramble
- 1 (14-ounce) can black beans
- 1/4 cup nutritional yeast
- 2 teaspoons hot sauce
- 10 small corn tortillas
- 1/2 cup shredded vegan Cheddar or pepper Jack cheese, divided

Directions:
1. Preheat the oven to 350°F. Coat a 9-by-9-inch baking pan with cooking spray.
2. In a large bowl, combine the tofu scramble with the black beans, nutritional yeast, and hot sauce. Set aside.
3. In the bottom of the baking pan, place 5 corn tortillas. Spread half of the tofu and bean mixture over the tortillas. Spread 1/4 cup of cheese over the

top. Layer the remaining 5 tortillas over the top of the cheese. Spread the reminder of the tofu and bean mixture over the tortillas. Spread the remaining 1/4 cup of cheese over the top.
4. Bake for 20 minutes.
5. Divide evenly among 6 single-serving containers. Let cool before sealing the lids.

Nutrition:

Calories: 132;

Fat: 10g;

Protein: 34g;

Carbohydrates: 54g;

Fiber: 9g;

Sugar: 4g;

Sodium: 254mg

Tofu-Spinach Scramble

Preparation Time: 15 minutes

Cooking time: 20minutes

Servings: 5

Ingredients:

- 1 (14-ounce) package water-packed extra-firm tofu
- 1 teaspoon extra-virgin olive oil or 1/4 cup vegetable broth
- 1 small yellow onion, diced
- 3 teaspoons minced garlic (about 3 cloves)
- 3 large celery stalks, chopped
- 2 large carrots, peeled (optional) and chopped
- 1 teaspoon chili powder
- 1/2 teaspoon ground cumin
- 1/2 teaspoon ground turmeric
- 1/2 teaspoon salt (optional)
- 1/4 teaspoon freshly ground black pepper
- 5 cups loosely packed spinach

Directions:

1. Drain the tofu by placing it, wrapped in a paper towel, on a plate in the sink. Place a cutting board over the tofu, then set a heavy pot, can, or cookbook

on the cutting board. Remove after 10 minutes. (Alternatively, use a tofu press.)

2. In a medium bowl, crumble the tofu with your hands or a potato masher.
3. Heat the olive oil. Add the onion, garlic, celery, and carrots, and sauté for 5 minutes, until the onion is softened.
4. Add the crumbled tofu, chili powder, cumin, turmeric, salt (if using), and pepper, and continue cooking for 7 to 8 more minutes, stirring frequently, until the tofu begins to brown.
5. Add the spinach and mix well. Cover and reduce the heat to medium. Steam the spinach for 3 minutes.
6. Divide evenly among 5 single-serving containers. Let cool before sealing the lids.

Nutrition:
Calories: 122;
Fat: 15g;
Protein: 14g;
Carbohydrates: 54g;
Fiber: 8g;
Sugar: 1g;
Sodium: 354mg

Savory Pancakes

Preparation Time: 10 minutes

Cooking time: 15minutes

Servings: 4

Ingredients:

- 1 cup whole-wheat flour
- 1 teaspoon garlic salt
- 1 teaspoon onion powder
- 1/2 teaspoon baking soda
- 1/4 teaspoon salt
- 1 cup lightly pressed, crumbled soft or firm tofu
- 1/2 cup unsweetened plant-based milk
- 1/4 cup lemon juice
- 2 tablespoons extra-virgin olive oil
- 1/2 cup finely chopped mushrooms
- 1/2 cup finely chopped onion
- 2 cups tightly packed greens (arugula, spinach, or baby kale work great)

Directions:

1. Attach the flour, garlic salt, onion powder, baking soda, and salt. Mix well. In a blender, combine the

tofu, plant-based milk, lemon juice, and olive oil. Purée on high speed for 30 seconds.
2. Pour the contents of the blender into the bowl of dry ingredients and whisk until combined well. Fold in the mushrooms, onion, and greens.

Nutrition:

Calories: 132;

Fat: 10g;

Protein: 12g;

Carbohydrates: 44g;

Fiber: 9g;

Sugar: 1g;

Sodium: 254mg

Quinoa Breakfast Porridge

Preparation Time: 10 minutes

Cooking time: 5 minutes

Servings: 3

Ingredients:

- 1 cup dry quinoa
- 2 cups almond milk
- 1 tbsp. agave or maple syrup
- 1/2 tsp. vanilla
- 1/2 tsp. cinnamon
- 1 tablespoon ground flax meal

Directions:

1. Combine quinoa, almond milk, sugar, vanilla, and cinnamon in a little pot. Heat to the point of boiling and lessen to a stew.
2. Allow the quinoa to cook until the majority of the fluid is retained, and quinoa is fleecy (15-20 minutes). Blend in the flax meal. Blend in any extra toppers or include INS, and appreciate.

Nutrition:

Calories: 122;

Fat: 12g;

Protein: 12g;

Carbohydrates: 34g;

Fiber: 9g;

Sugar: 5g;

Sodium: 154mg

Grapes and Green Tea Smoothie

Preparation Time: 5 Minutes
Cooking Time: 0 Minutes
Servings: 2

Ingredients:

- ½ cup green tea
- ½ cup of green grapes
- 1 banana, peeled
- 1-inch piece of ginger
- ½ cup of ice cubes
- 2 cups baby spinach
- ½ of a medium apple, peeled, diced

Directions:

1. Place all the ingredients into the jar of a high-speed food processor or blender in the order stated in the ingredients list and then cover it with the lid.
2. Pulse for 1 minute until smooth, and then serve.

Nutrition:

Calories: 150 Cal;

Fat: 2.5 g;

Protein: 1 g;

Carbs: 36.5 g;
Fiber: 9 g

Mango and Kale Smoothie

Preparation Time: 5 Minutes
Cooking Time: 0 Minutes
Servings: 2

Ingredients:

- 2 cups oats milk, unsweetened
- 2 bananas, peeled
- ½ cup kale leaves
- 2 teaspoons coconut sugar
- 1 cup mango pieces
- 1 teaspoon vanilla extract, unsweetened

Directions:

1. Place all the ingredients into the jar of a high-speed food processor or blender in the order stated in the ingredients list and then cover it with the lid.
2. Pulse for 1 minute until smooth, and then serve.

Nutrition:

Calories: 281 Cal;

Fat: 3 g;

Protein: 6 g;

Carbs: 63 g;

Fiber: 16 g

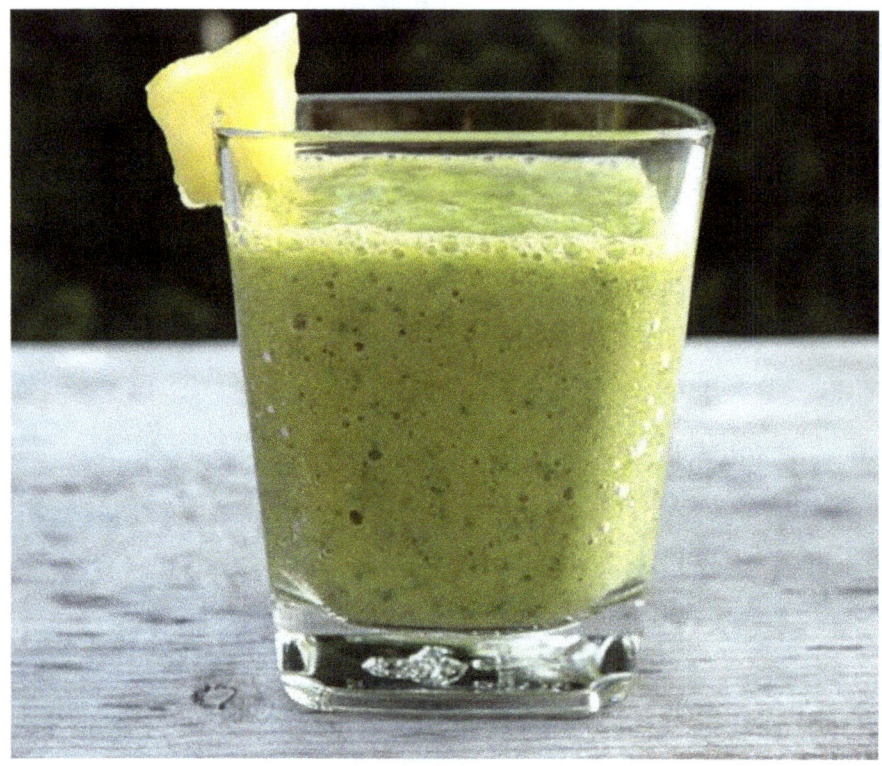

Pomegranate Smoothie

Preparation Time: 5 Minutes
Cooking Time: 0 Minutes
Servings: 2

Ingredients:

- 2 cups almond milk, unsweetened
- 2 medium apples, cored, sliced
- 2 bananas, peeled
- 2 cups frozen raspberries
- 1 cup pomegranate seeds
- 4 teaspoons agave syrup

Directions:

1. Place all the ingredients into the jar of a high-speed food processor or blender in the order stated in the ingredients list and then cover it with the lid.
2. Pulse for 1 minute until smooth, and then serve.

Nutrition:
Calories: 141.5 Cal;
Fat: 1.1 g;
Protein: 4.1 g;
Carbs: 30.8 g;

Fiber: 2.4 g

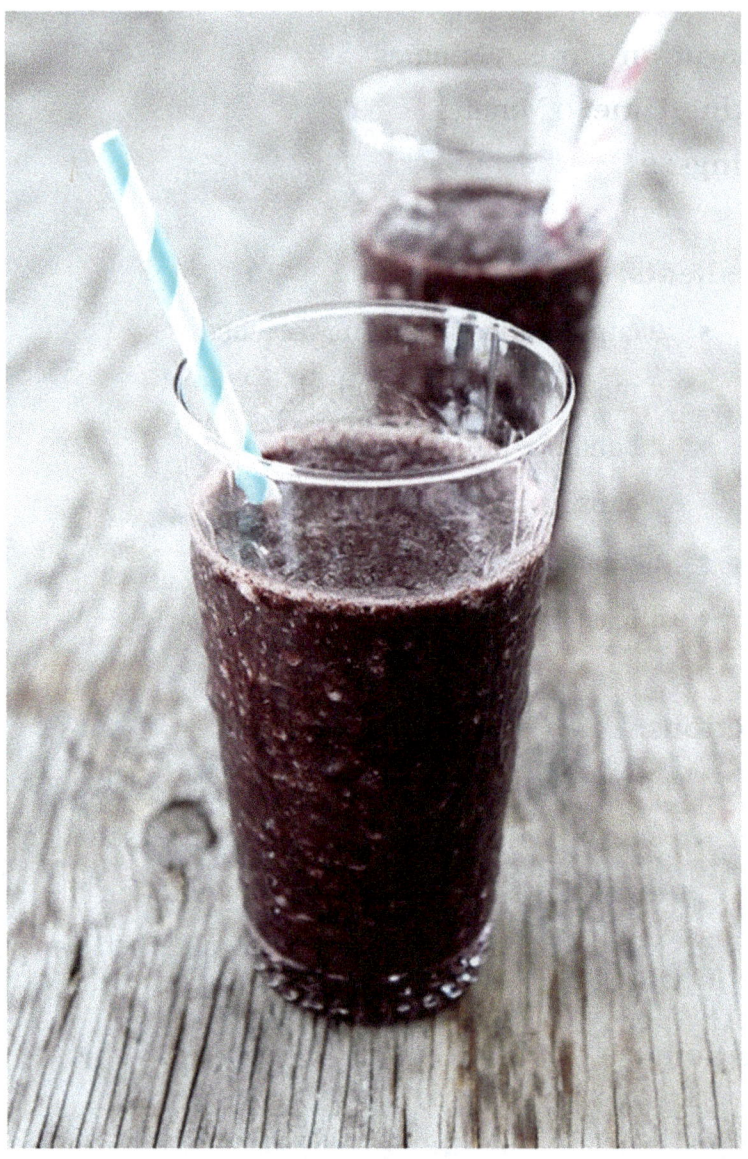

Coconut Water Smoothie

Preparation Time: 5 Minutes
Cooking Time: 0 Minutes
Servings: 2

Ingredients:

- 2 cups of coconut water
- 1 large apple, peeled, cored, diced
- 1 cup of frozen mango pieces
- 2 teaspoons peanut butter
- 4 teaspoons coconut flakes

Directions:

1. Place all the ingredients into the jar of a high-speed food processor or blender in the order stated in the ingredients list and then cover it with the lid.
2. Pulse for 1 minute until smooth, and then serve.

Nutrition:
Calories: 113.4 Cal;
Fat: 0.3 g;
Protein: 0.6 g;
Carbs: 29 g;
Fiber: 2 g

Apple, Banana, and Berry Smoothie

Preparation Time: 5 Minutes

Cooking Time: 0 Minutes

Servings: 2

Ingredients:

- 2 cups almond milk, unsweetened
- 2 cups frozen strawberries
- 2 bananas, peeled
- 1 large apple, peeled, cored, diced
- 2 tablespoons peanut butter

Directions:

1. Place all the ingredients into the jar of a high-speed food processor or blender in the order stated in the ingredients list and then cover it with the lid.
2. Pulse for 1 minute until smooth, and then serve.

Nutrition:

Calories: 156.1 Cal;

Fat: 3.2 g;

Protein: 3 g;

Carbs: 17 g;

Fiber: 5.8 g

Berry Ginger Zing Smoothie

Preparation Time: 5 Minutes

Cooking Time: 0 Minutes

Servings: 2

Ingredients:

- 2 cups almond milk, unsweetened
- 1 cup frozen raspberries
- 1 cup of frozen strawberries
- 1 cup cauliflower florets
- 1-inch pieces of ginger

Directions:

1. Place all the ingredients into the jar of a high-speed food processor or blender in the order stated in the ingredients list and then cover it with the lid.
2. Pulse for 1 minute until smooth, and then serve.

Nutrition:

Calories: 300 Cal;

Fat: 8 g;

Protein: 8 g;

Carbs: 30 g;

Fiber: 9 g

Dragon Fruit Smoothie Bowl

Preparation Time: 5 Minutes

Cooking Time: 0 Minutes

Servings: 2

Ingredients:

For the Bowl:

- ½ cup coconut milk, unsweetened
- 2 bananas, peeled
- ½ cup frozen raspberries
- 7 ounces frozen dragon fruit
- 3 tablespoons vanilla protein powder

For the Toppings:

- 2 tablespoons coconut flakes
- 2 tablespoons hemp seeds

Directions:

1. Place all the ingredients for the bowl into the jar of a high-speed food processor or blender in the order stated in the ingredients list and then cover it with the lid.

2. Pulse for 1 minute until smooth, and then divide evenly between two bowls.

3. Sprinkle 1 tablespoon of coconut flakes and hemp seeds over the smoothie and then serve.

Nutrition:

Calories: 225 Cal;

Fat: 1.6 g;

Protein: 8.1 g;

Carbs: 48 g;

Fiber: 8.9 g

Chocolate Smoothie Bowl

Preparation Time: 5 Minutes

Cooking Time: 0 Minutes

Servings: 2

Ingredients:

For the Bowls:

- 2 cups almond milk, unsweetened
- 2 bananas, peeled
- 3 tablespoons cocoa powder
- 1 cup spinach leaves, fresh
- 2 tablespoons oat flour
- 4 Medjool dates, pitted
- 1/8 teaspoon salt
- 2 tablespoons vanilla protein powder
- 2 tablespoons peanut butter

For the Toppings:

- 2 tablespoons coconut flakes
- 2 tablespoons hemp seeds

Directions:

1. Place all the ingredients for the bowl into the jar of a high-speed food processor or blender in the order stated in the ingredients list and then cover it with the lid.
2. Pulse for 1 minute until smooth, and then divide evenly between two bowls.
3. Sprinkle 1 tablespoon of coconut flakes and hemp seeds over the smoothie and then serve.

Nutrition:

Calories: 382 Cal;

Fat: 14 g;

Protein: 22 g;

Carbs: 53 g;

Fiber: 9 g

Zucchini and Blueberry Smoothie

Preparation Time: 5 Minutes

Cooking Time: 0 Minutes

Servings: 2

Ingredients:

- 1 cup coconut milk, unsweetened
- 1 large celery stem
- 2 bananas, peeled
- ½ cup spinach leaves, fresh
- 1 cup frozen blueberries
- 2/3 cup sliced zucchini
- 1 tablespoon hemp seeds
- ½ teaspoon maca powder
- ¼ teaspoon ground cinnamon

Directions:

1. Place all the ingredients into the jar of a high-speed food processor or blender in the order stated in the ingredients list and then cover it with the lid.
2. Pulse for 1 minute until smooth, and then serve.

Nutrition:

Calories: 218 Cal;

Fat: 10.1 g;

Protein: 6.3 g;

Carbs: 31.8 g;

Fiber: 4.7 g

Hot Pink Beet Smoothie

Preparation Time: 5 Minutes

Cooking Time: 0 Minutes

Servings: 2

Ingredients:

- 2 cups almond milk, unsweetened
- 2 clementine, peeled
- 1 cup raspberries
- 1 banana, peeled
- 1 medium beet, peeled, chopped
- 2 tablespoons chia seeds
- 1/8 teaspoon sea salt
- ½ teaspoon vanilla extract, unsweetened
- 4 tablespoons almond butter

Directions:

1. Place all the ingredients into the jar of a high-speed food processor or blender in the order stated in the ingredients list and then cover it with the lid.
2. Pulse for 1 minute until smooth, and then serve.

Nutrition:

Calories: 260.8 Cal;

Fat: 1.3 g;

Protein: 13 g;

Carbs: 56 g;

Fiber: 9.3 g

Chickpea Flour Frittata

Preparation Time: 10 Minutes

Cooking Time: 50 Minutes

Servings: 6

Ingredients:

- 1 medium green bell pepper, cored, chopped
- 1 cup chopped greens
- 1 cup cauliflower florets, chopped
- ½ cup chopped broccoli florets
- ½ of a medium red onion, peeled, chopped
- ¼ teaspoon salt
- ½ cup chopped zucchini

For the Batter:

- ¼ cup cashew cream
- ½ cup chickpea flour

- ½ cup chopped cilantro

- ½ teaspoon salt

- ¼ teaspoon cayenne pepper

- ½ teaspoon dried dill

- ¼ teaspoon ground black pepper

- ¼ teaspoon dried thyme

- ½ teaspoon ground turmeric

- 1 tablespoon olive oil

- 1 ½ cup water

Directions:

1. Switch on the oven, then set it to 375 degrees F and let it preheat.

2. Take a 9-inch pie pan, grease it with oil, and then set aside until required.

3. Take a large bowl, place all the vegetables in it, sprinkle with salt and then toss until combined.

4. Prepare the batter and for this, add all of its ingredients in it except for thyme, dill, and cilantro and then pulse until combined and smooth.

5. Pour the batter over the vegetables, add dill, thyme, and cilantro, and then stir until combined.

6. Spoon the mixture into the prepared pan, spread evenly, and then bake for 45 to 50 minutes until done and inserted toothpick into frittata comes out clean.

7. When done, let the frittata rest for 10 minutes, cut it into slices, and then serve.

Nutrition:

Calories: 153 Cal;

Fat: 4 g;

Protein: 7 g;

Carbs: 20 g;

Fiber: 4 g

Potato Pancakes

Preparation Time: 10 Minutes

Cooking Time: 20 Minutes

Servings: 10

Ingredients:

- ½ cup white whole-wheat flour
- 3 large potatoes, grated
- ½ of a medium white onion, peeled, grated
- 1 jalapeno, minced
- 2 green onions, chopped
- 1 tablespoon minced garlic
- 1 teaspoon salt
- ¼ teaspoon baking powder
- ¼ teaspoon ground pepper
- 4 tablespoons olive oil

Directions:

1. Take a large bowl, place all the ingredients except for oil and then stir until well combined; stir in 1 to 2 tablespoons water if needed to mix the batter.

2. Take a large skillet pan, place it over medium-high heat, add 2 tablespoons of oil and then let it heat.

3. Scoop the pancake mixture in portions into the pan, shape each portion like a pancake and then cook for 5 to 7 minutes per side until pancakes turn golden brown and thoroughly cooked.

4. When done, transfer the pancakes to a plate, add more oil into the pan and then cook more pancakes in the same manner.

5. Serve straight away.

Nutrition:

Calories: 69 Cal;

Fat: 1 g;

Protein: 2 g;

Carbs: 12 g;

Fiber: 1 g

Chocolate Chip Pancakes

Preparation Time: 5 Minutes

Cooking Time: 10 Minutes

Servings: 6

Ingredients:

- 1 cup white whole-wheat flour
- ½ cup chocolate chips, vegan, unsweetened
- 1 tablespoon baking powder
- ¼ teaspoon salt
- 2 teaspoons coconut sugar
- ½ teaspoon vanilla extract, unsweetened
- 1 cup almond milk, unsweetened
- 2 tablespoons coconut butter, melted
- 2 tablespoons olive oil

Directions:

1. Take a large bowl, place all the ingredients except for oil and chocolate chips, and then stir until well combined.

2. Add chocolate chips, and then fold until just mixed.

3. Take a large skillet pan, place it over medium-high heat, add 1 tablespoon oil and then let it heat.

4. Scoop the pancake mixture in portions into the pan, shape each portion like a pancake and then cook for 5 to 7 minutes per side until pancakes turn golden brown and thoroughly cooked.

5. When done, transfer the pancakes to a plate, add more oil into the pan and then cook more pancakes in the same manner.

6. Serve straight away.

Nutrition:

Calories: 172 Cal;
Fat: 6 g;
Protein: 2.5 g;
Carbs: 28 g;
Fiber: 8 g

Turmeric Steel-Cut Oats

Preparation Time: 5 Minutes

Cooking Time: 10 Minutes

Servings: 2

Ingredients:

- ½ cup steel-cut oats
- 1/8 teaspoon salt
- 2 tablespoons maple syrup
- ½ teaspoon ground cinnamon
- 1/3 teaspoon turmeric powder
- ¼ teaspoon ground cardamom
- ¼ teaspoon olive oil
- ½ cups water
- 1 cup almond milk, unsweetened

For the Topping:

- 2 tablespoons pumpkin seeds
- 2 tablespoons chia seeds

Directions:

1. Take a medium saucepan, place it over medium heat, add oats, and then cook for 2 minutes until toasted.
2. Pour in the milk and water, stir until mixed, and then bring the oats to a boil.
3. Then switch heat to medium-low level, simmer the oats for 10 minutes, and add salt, maple syrup, and all spices.
4. Stir until combined, cook the oats for 7 minutes or more until cooked to the desired level and when done, let the oats rest for 15 minutes.
5. When done, divide oats evenly between two bowls, top with pumpkin seeds and chia seeds and then serve.

Nutrition:

Calories: 234 Cal;

Fat: 4 g;

Protein: 7 g;

Carbs: 41 g;
Fiber: 5 g

Vegetable Pancakes

Preparation Time: 10 Minutes

Cooking Time: 20 Minutes

Servings: 10

Ingredients:

- 1/3 cup cooked and mashed sweet potato
- 2 cups grated carrots
- 1 cup chopped coriander
- 1 cup cooked spinach
- 2 ounces chickpea flour
- ½ teaspoon baking powder
- 1 ½ teaspoon salt
- 1 teaspoon ground turmeric
- 2 tablespoons olive oil
- ¾ cup of water

Directions:

1. Take a large bowl, place chickpea flour in it, add turmeric powder, baking powder, and salt, and then stir until combined.

2. Whisk in the water until combined, stir in sweet potatoes until well mixed and then add carrots, spinach, and coriander until well combined.

3. Take a large skillet pan, place it over medium-high heat, add 1 tablespoon oil and then let it heat.

4. Scoop the pancake mixture in portions into the pan, shape each portion like a pancake and then cook for 3 to 5 minutes per side until pancakes turn golden brown and thoroughly cooked.

5. When done, transfer the pancakes to a plate, add more oil into the pan and then cook more pancakes in the same manner.

6. Serve straight away.

Nutrition:

Calories: 74 Cal;

Fat: 0.3 g;

Protein: 3 g;

Carbs: 16 g;

Fiber: 2.7 g

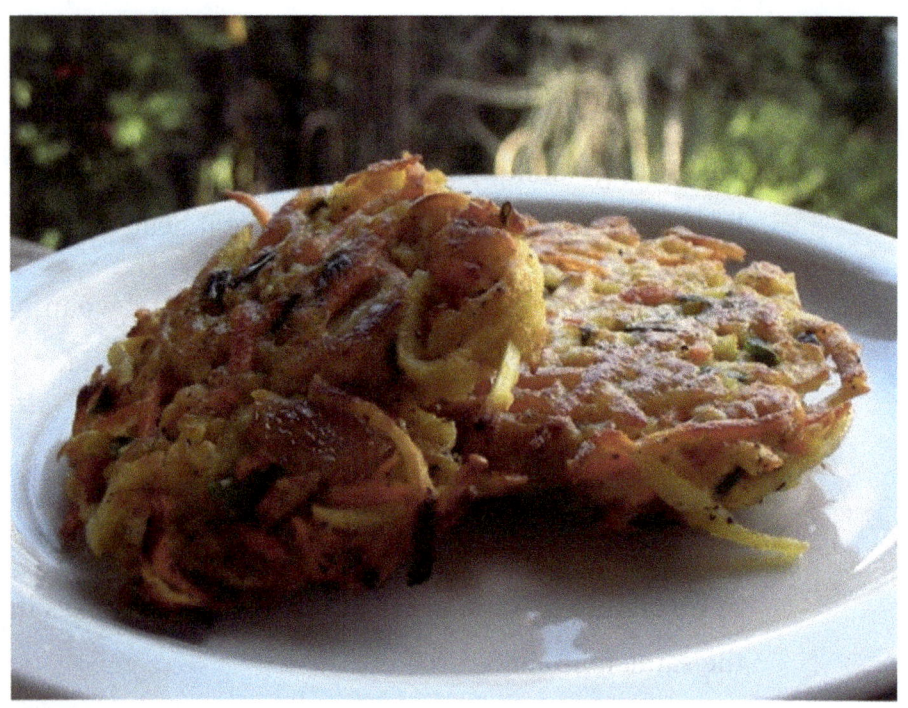

Banana and Chia Pudding

Preparation Time: 25 Minutes

Cooking Time: 12 Minutes

Servings: 2

Ingredients:

For the Pudding:

- 2 bananas, peeled
- 4 tablespoons chia seeds
- 2 tablespoons coconut sugar
- ½ teaspoon pumpkin pie spice
- 1/8 teaspoon sea salt
- ½ cup almond milk, unsweetened

For the Bananas:

- 2 bananas, peeled, sliced
- 2 tablespoons coconut flakes

- 1/8 teaspoon ground cinnamon
- 2 tablespoons coconut sugar
- ¼ cup chopped walnuts
- 2 tablespoons almond milk, unsweetened

Directions:

1. Prepare the pudding and for this, place all of its ingredients in a blender except for chia seeds and then pulse until smooth.

2. Pour the mixture into a medium saucepan, place it over medium heat, bring the mixture to a boil and then remove the pan from heat.

3. Add chia seeds into the hot banana mixture, stir until mixed, and then let it sit for 5 minutes.

4. Whisk the pudding and then let it chill for 15 minutes in the refrigerator.

5. Meanwhile, prepare the caramelized bananas and for this, take a medium skillet pan, and place it over medium heat.

6. Add banana slices, sprinkle with salt, sugar, and nutmeg, drizzle with milk and then cook for 5 minutes until mixture has thickened.

7. Assemble the pudding and for this, divide the pudding evenly between two bowls, top with banana slices, sprinkle with walnuts, and then serve.

Nutrition:

Calories: 495 Cal;

Fat: 21 g;

Protein: 9 g;

Carbs: 76 g;

Fiber: 14 g

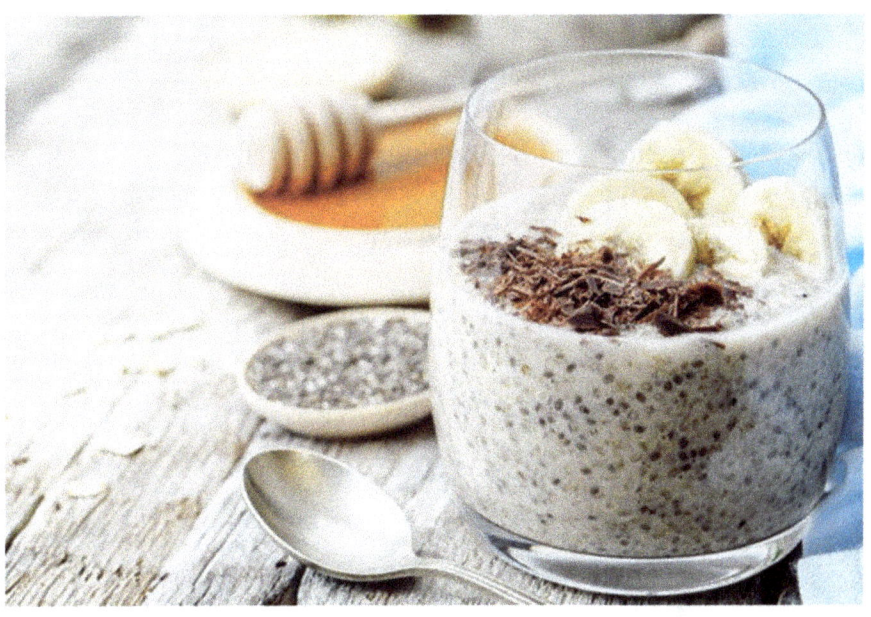

Tofu Scramble

Preparation Time: 5 Minutes

Cooking Time: 15 Minutes

Servings: 3

Ingredients:

- 12 ounces tofu, extra-firm, pressed, drained
- ½ of a medium red onion, peeled, sliced
- 1 cup baby greens mix
- 1 medium red bell pepper, cored, sliced
- ½ teaspoon garlic powder
- 1 teaspoon salt
- ½ teaspoon ground black pepper
- ¼ teaspoon turmeric powder
- ¼ teaspoon ground cumin
- 4 tablespoons olive oil, divided

Directions:

1. Take a large bowl, place tofu in it, and then break it into bite-size pieces.

2. Add salt, black pepper, turmeric, and 2 tablespoons of oil, and then stir until mixed.

3. Take a medium skillet pan, place it over medium heat, add garlic powder and cumin and then cook for 1 minute until fragrant.

4. Add tofu mixture, stir until mixed, switch heat to medium-high level, and then cook for 5 minutes until tofu turn golden brown.

5. When done, divide tofu evenly between three plates, keep it warm, and then set aside until required.

6. Return the skillet pan over medium-high heat, add remaining oil and let it heat until hot.

7. Add onion and bell peppers, cook for 5 to 7 minutes or until beginning to brown, and then season with a pinch of salt.

8. Add baby greens, toss until mixed, and then cook for 30 seconds until leaves begin to wilts.

9. Add vegetables evenly to the plates to scrambled tofu and then serve.

Nutrition:

Calories: 304 Cal;

Fat: 25.6 g;

Protein: 14.2 g;

Carbs: 6.6 g;

Fiber: 2.6 g

Pumpkin Spice Oatmeal

Preparation Time: 5 Minutes

Cooking Time: 8 Minutes

Servings: 2

Ingredients:

- ¼ cup Medjool dates, pitted, chopped
- 2/3 cup rolled oats
- 1 tablespoon maple syrup
- ½ teaspoon pumpkin pie spice
- ½ teaspoon vanilla extract, unsweetened
- 1/3 cup pumpkin puree
- 2 tablespoons chopped pecans
- 1 cup almond milk, unsweetened

Directions:

1. Take a medium pot, place it over medium heat, and then add all the ingredients except for pecans and maple syrup.

2. Stir all the ingredients until combined, and then cook for 5 minutes until the oatmeal has absorbed all the liquid and thickened to the desired level.

3. When done, divide oatmeal evenly between two bowls, top with pecans, drizzle with maple syrup and then serve.

Nutrition:

Calories: 175 Cal;

Fat: 3.2 g;

Protein: 5.8 g;

Carbs: 33 g;

Fiber: 6.1 g

Peanut Butter Bites

Preparation Time: 10 Minutes

Cooking Time: 0 Minutes

Servings: 5

Ingredients:

- 1 cup rolled oats
- 12 Medjool dates, pitted
- ½ cup peanut butter, sugar-free

Directions:

1. Plug in a blender or a food processor, add all the ingredients in its jar, and then cover with the lid.
2. Pulse for 5 minutes until well combined, and then tip the mixture into a shallow dish.
3. Shape the mixture into 20 balls, 1 tablespoon of mixture per ball, and then serve.

Nutrition:

Calories: 103.1 Cal;

Fat: 4.3 g;

Protein: 2.3 g;

Carbs: 15.4 g;

Fiber: 0.8 g

Maple and Cinnamon Overnight Oats

Preparation Time: 10 Minutes

Cooking Time: 0 Minutes

Servings: 4

Ingredients:

- 2 cups rolled oats
- ¼ cup chopped pecans
- ¾ teaspoon ground cinnamon
- 1 teaspoon vanilla extract, unsweetened
- 3 tablespoons coconut sugar
- 3 tablespoons maple syrup
- 2 cups almond milk, unsweetened

Directions:

1. Take four mason jars, and then add ½ cup oats, ¼ teaspoon vanilla, and ½ cup milk.

2. Take a small bowl, add maple syrup, cinnamon, and sugar, stir until mixed, add this mixture into the oats mixture and then stir until combined.

3. Cover the jars with the lid and then let them rest in the refrigerator for a minimum of 2 hours or more until thickened.

4. When ready to eat, top the oats with pecans, sprinkle with cinnamon, drizzle with maple syrup and then serve.

Nutrition:

Calories: 292 Cal;

Fat: 9 g;

Protein: 7 g;

Carbs: 48 g;

Fiber: 6 g

Breakfast Tomato and Eggs

Preparation Time: 5 Minutes

Cooking Time: 30 Minutes

Servings: 2

Ingredients:

- 2 eggs
- 2 tomatoes
- Salt and black pepper to taste
- 1 tsp. parsley, finely chopped

Directions:

1. Cut tomatoes tops, scoop flesh and arrange them on a lined baking sheet.

2. Crack an egg in each tomato.

3. Season with salt and pepper.

4. Introduce them in the oven at 150 degrees and bake for 30 minutes

5. Take tomatoes out of the oven, divide between plates, season with more salt and pepper, sprinkle parsley at the end and serve.

6. Enjoy!

Nutrition:

Calories: 186

Fat: 36g

Carbs: 2g

Protein: 14g

Fiber: 11.6g

Sugar: 0g

Breakfast Paleo Muffins

Preparation Time: 5 Minutes

Cooking Time: 30 Minutes

Servings: 4

Ingredients:

- 1 cup kale, chopped
- ¼ cup chives, finely chopped
- ½ cup almond milk
- 6 eggs
- Salt and black pepper to taste
- Some coconut oil for greasing the muffin cups

Directions:

1. In a bowl, mix eggs with chives and kale and whisk very well.

2. Add salt and black pepper to the taste and almond milk and stir well.

3. Divide this into eight muffin cups after you've greased it with some coconut oil.

4. Introduce this in preheated oven at 150 degrees and bake for 30 minutes

5. Take muffins out of the oven, leave them to cool down, transfer them to plates and serve warm.

6. Enjoy!

Nutrition:

Calories: 100

Fat: 5g

Carbs: 3g

Protein: 14g

Fiber: 10.6g

Sugar: 0g

Paleo Banana Pancakes

Preparation Time: 5 Minutes

Cooking Time: 5 Minutes

Servings: 2

Ingredients:

- 4 eggs
- A pinch of salt
- Two bananas, peeled and chopped
- ¼ tsp. baking powder
- Cooking spray

Directions:

1. In a bowl, mix eggs with chopped bananas, a pinch of salt and baking powder and whisk well.

2. Transfer this to your food processor and blend very well.

3. Heat up a pan over medium high heat after you've sprayed it with some cooking oil.

4. Add some of the pancakes batter, spread in the pan, cook for

1 minute, flip and cook for 30 seconds and transfer to a plate.

5. Serve and enjoy!

Nutrition:

Calories: 120

Fat: 2g

Carbs: 2g

Protein: 4g

Fiber: 6.6g

Sugar: 1g

Breakfast Eggs

Preparation Time: 5 Minutes

Cooking Time: 30 Minutes

Servings: 2

Ingredients:

- 2 eggs
- Salt and black pepper to taste
- 1 tsp. parsley, finely chopped

Directions:

1. Crack an egg in each tomato.

2. Season with salt and pepper.

3. Introduce them in the oven at 150 degrees and bake for 30 minutes

4. Divide between plates, season with more salt and pepper, sprinkle parsley at the end and serve.

5. Enjoy!

Nutrition:

Calories: 186

Fat: 10g

Carbs: 2g

Protein: 14g

Fiber: 6g

Sugar: 0g

Plantain Pancakes

Preparation Time: 5 Minutes

Cooking Time: 5 Minutes

Servings: 1

Ingredients:

- 3 eggs
- ¼ cup coconut flour
- ¼ cup coconut water
- 1 tsp. coconut oil
- ½ plantain, peeled and chopped
- ¼ tsp. cream of tartar
- ¼ tsp. baking soda
- A pinch of salt
- ¼ tsp. chai spice
- 1 tbsp. shaved coconut, toasted for serving

- 1 tbsp. coconut milk for serving

Directions:

1. In your food processor, mix eggs with a pinch of salt, coconut water and flour, plantain, cream of tartar, baking soda and chai spice and blend well.

2. Heat up a pan with the coconut oil over medium heat, add ¼ cup pancake batter, spread evenly, cook until it becomes golden, flip pancake and cook for one minute and transfer to a plate.

3. Serve pancakes with shaved coconut and coconut milk.

Nutrition:

Calories: 372

Fat: 17g

Carbs: 55g

Protein: 23g

Fiber: 5.6g

Sugar: 0g

Sweet Potato Waffles

Preparation Time: 5 Minutes

Cooking Time: 20 Minutes

Servings: 4

Ingredients:

- 2 sweet potatoes, peeled and finely grated
- 2 tbsp. melted coconut oil
- 3 eggs
- 1 tsp. cinnamon powder
- ½ tsp. nutmeg, ground
- Some apple sauce for serving

Directions:

1. In a bowl, mix eggs with sweet potatoes, coconut oil, cinnamon and nutmeg and whisk very well.
2. Cook waffles in your waffle iron, arrange them on plates and serve with apple sauce drizzled on top.
3. Enjoy!

Nutrition:

Calories: 227

Fat: 6g

Carbs: 37g

Protein: 6g

Fiber: 2g

Sugar: 2g

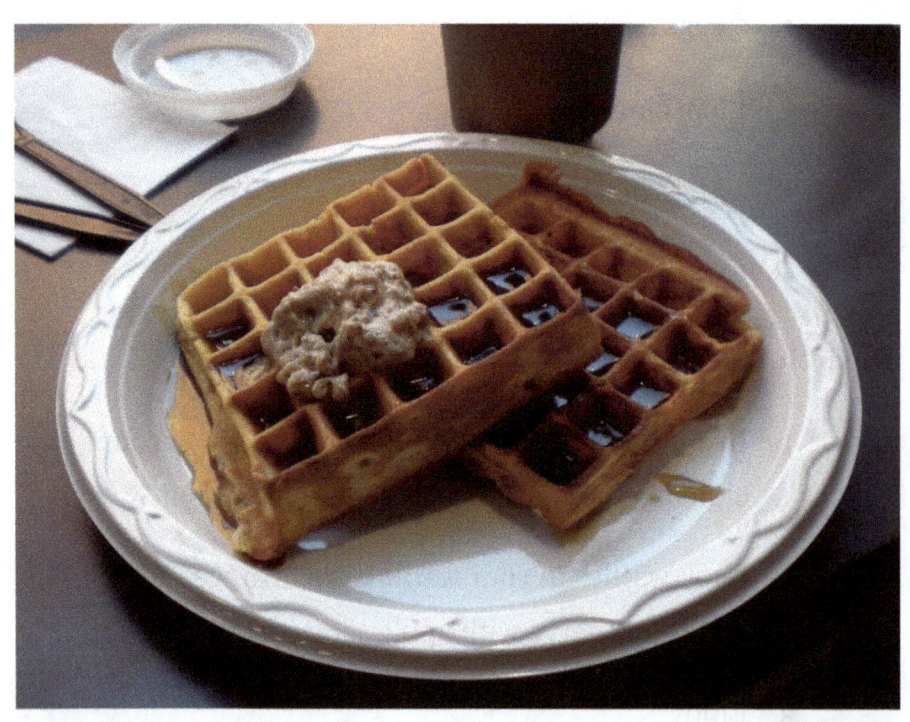

Eggplant French Toast

Preparation Time: 5 Minutes

Cooking Time: 5 Minutes

Servings: 2

Ingredients:

- 1 eggplant, peeled and sliced
- A pinch of sea salt
- 1 tsp. vanilla extract
- 2 eggs
- Stevia, to taste
- 1 tsp. coconut oil
- A pinch of cinnamon

Directions:

1. Arrange eggplant slices on a plate, sprinkle them with a pinch of salt, flip them and season with salt again and leave them aside for 2 minutes
2. In a bowl, mix eggs with vanilla, stevia, and cinnamon and whisk well.

3. Heat up a pan with the coconut oil over medium-high heat.

4. Dip eggplant slices in eggs mix, add to heated pan and cook until they become golden on each side.

5. Arrange them on plates and serve.

6. Enjoy!

Nutrition:

Calories: 125

Fat: 5g

Carbs: 13g

Protein: 7.8g

Fiber: 7.8g

Orange and Dates Granola

Preparation Time: 5 Minutes

Cooking Time: 25 Minutes

Servings: 6

Ingredients:

- 5 oz. dates, soaked in hot water
- Juice from 1 orange
- Grated rind of ½ orange
- 1 cup desiccated coconut
- ½ cup silvered almonds
- ½ cup pumpkin seeds
- ½ cup linseeds
- ½ cup sesame seeds
- Almond milk for serving

Directions:

1. In a bowl, mix almonds with orange rind, orange juice, linseeds, coconut, pumpkin and sesame seeds and stir well.
2. Drain dates, add them to your food processor and blend well.
3. Add this paste to almonds mix and stir well again.
4. Spread this on a lined baking sheet, introduce in the oven at 350 degrees and bake for 15 minutes, stirring every 4 minutes.
5. Take granola out of the oven, leave aside to cool down a bit and then serve with almond milk.
6. Enjoy!

Nutrition:

Calories: 208

Fat: 9g

Carbs: 3g

Protein: 6g

Fiber: 5g

Sugar: 0g

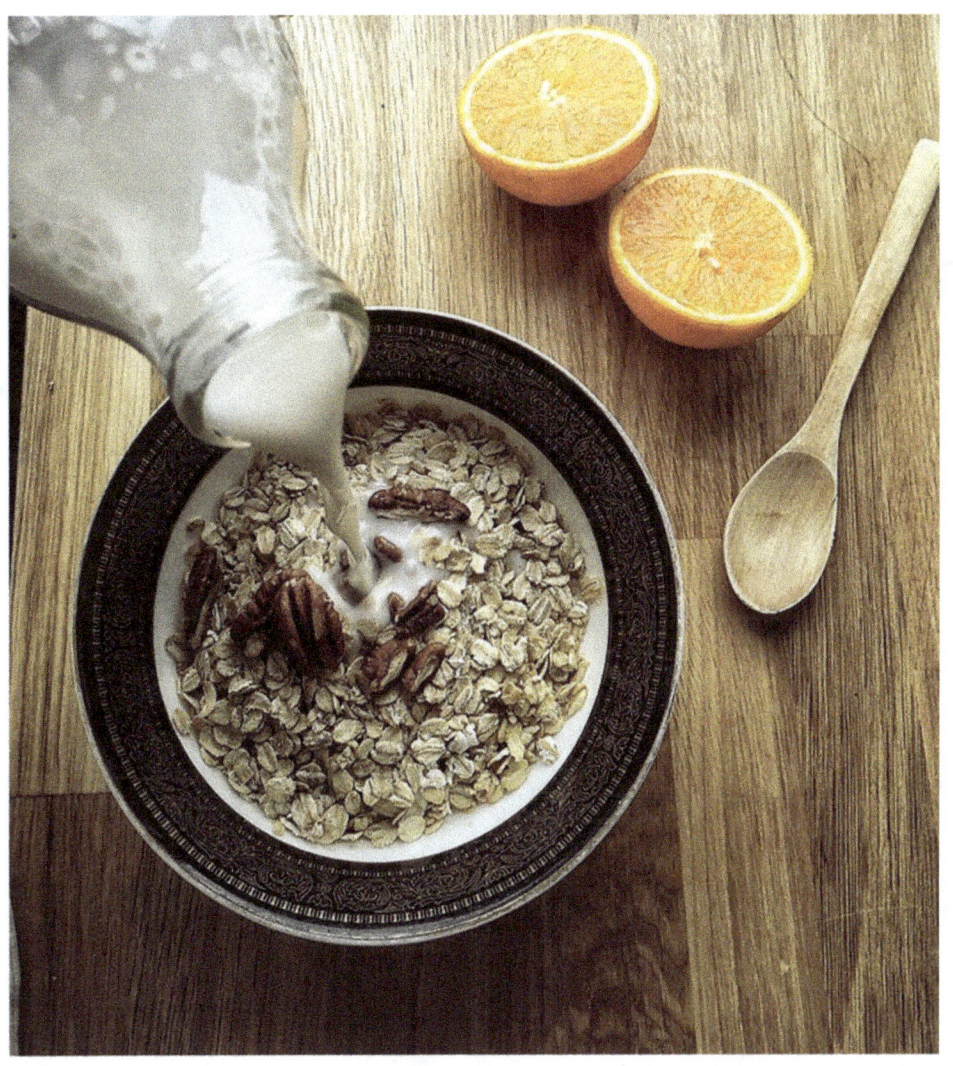

www.ingramcontent.com/pod-product-compliance
Lightning Source LLC
Chambersburg PA
CBHW070731030426
42336CB00013B/1939